THE DARK CLOUD OVER EMU'S HEAD

Dealing with DEPRESSION

Written & Illustrated by
Dr. Abraham Thomas

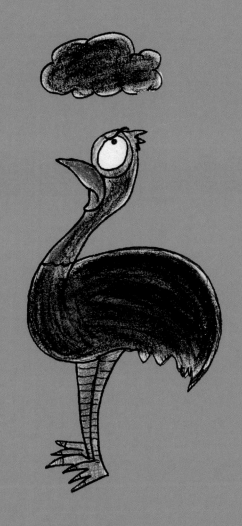

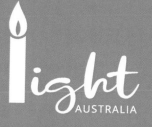

light
AUSTRALIA

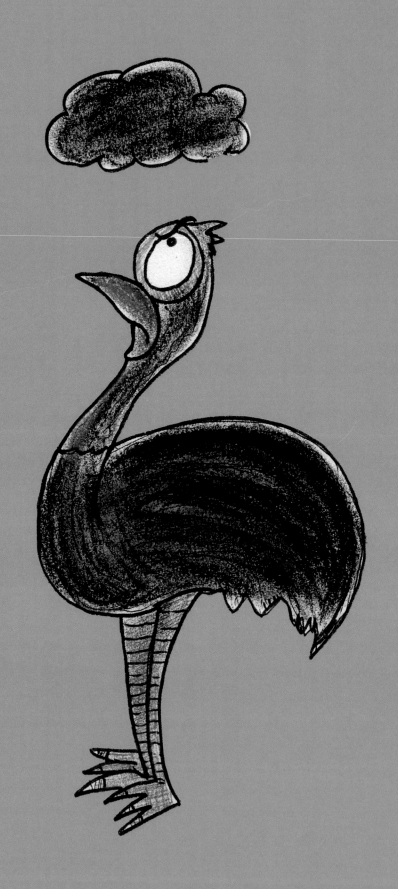

Today I can't see the sun as there is a
DARK CLOUD hanging over my head.

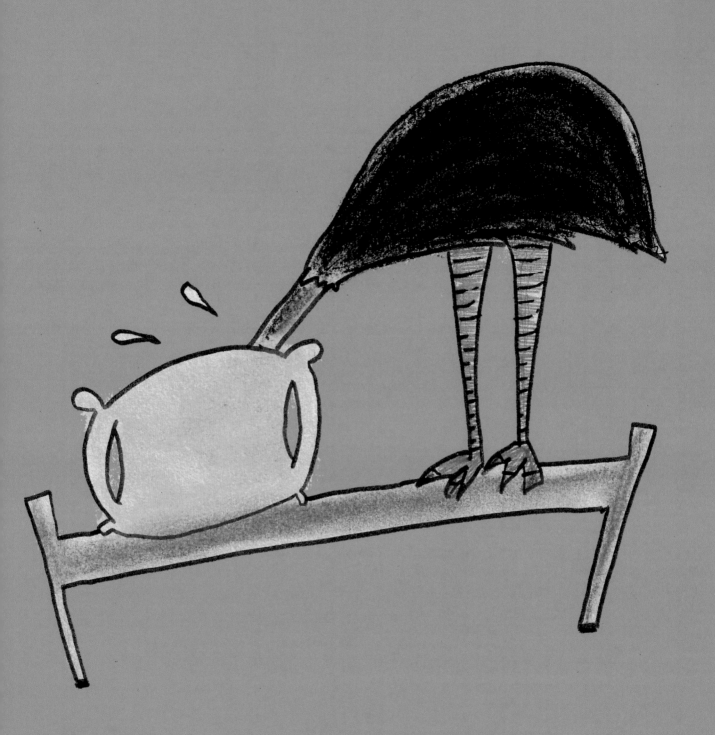

I felt like hiding my head under the pillow.

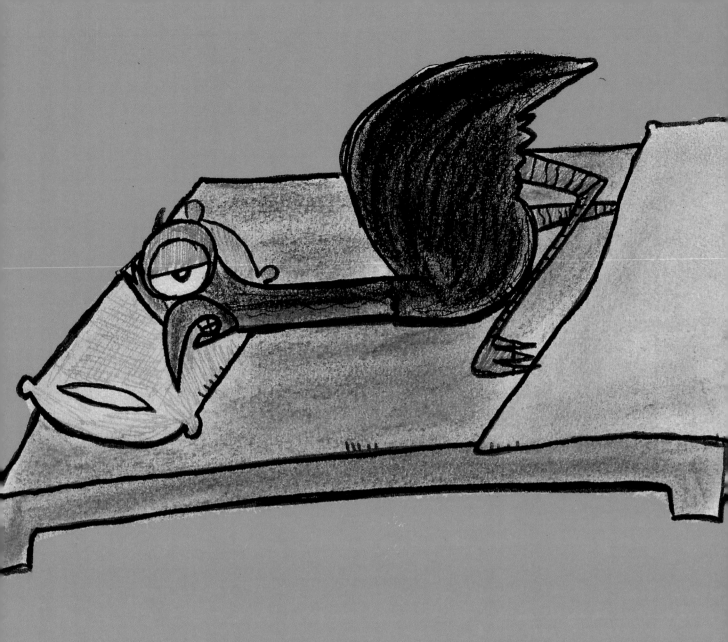

I didn't feel like getting up either.

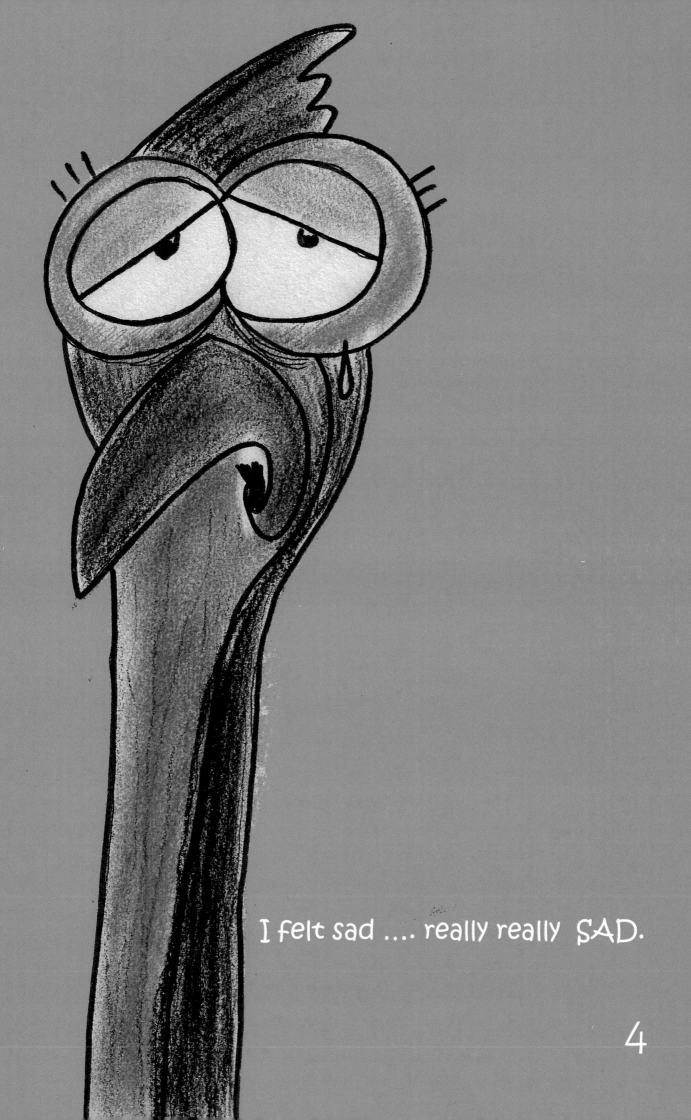

I felt sad .... really really SAD.

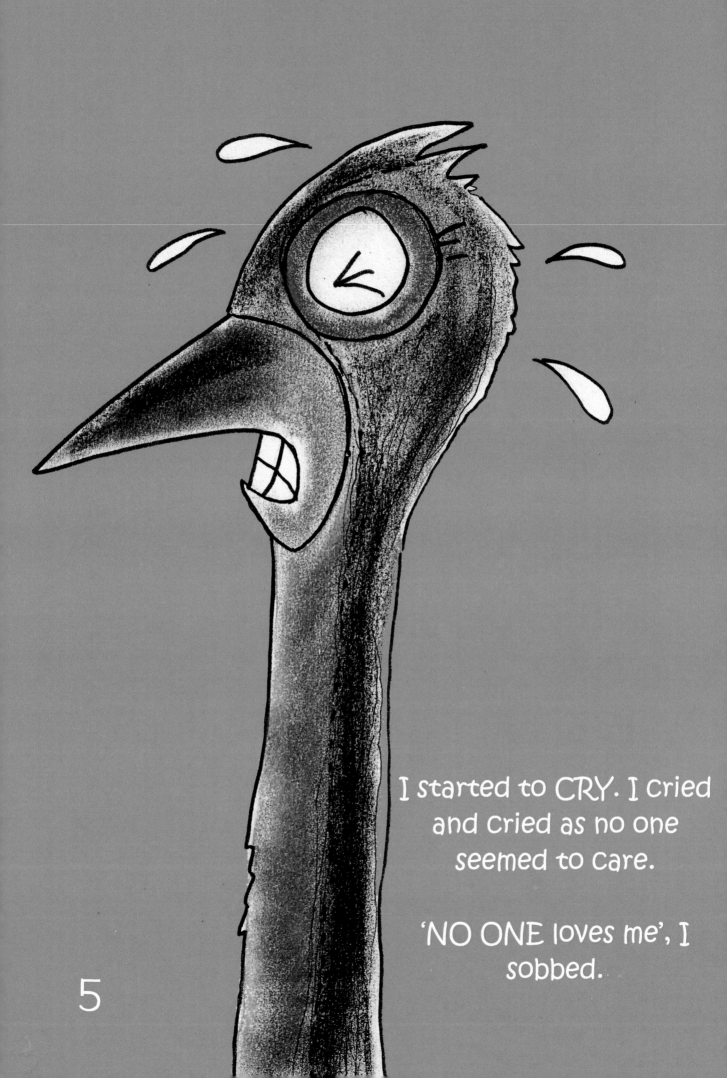

I started to CRY. I cried and cried as no one seemed to care.

'NO ONE loves me', I sobbed.

5

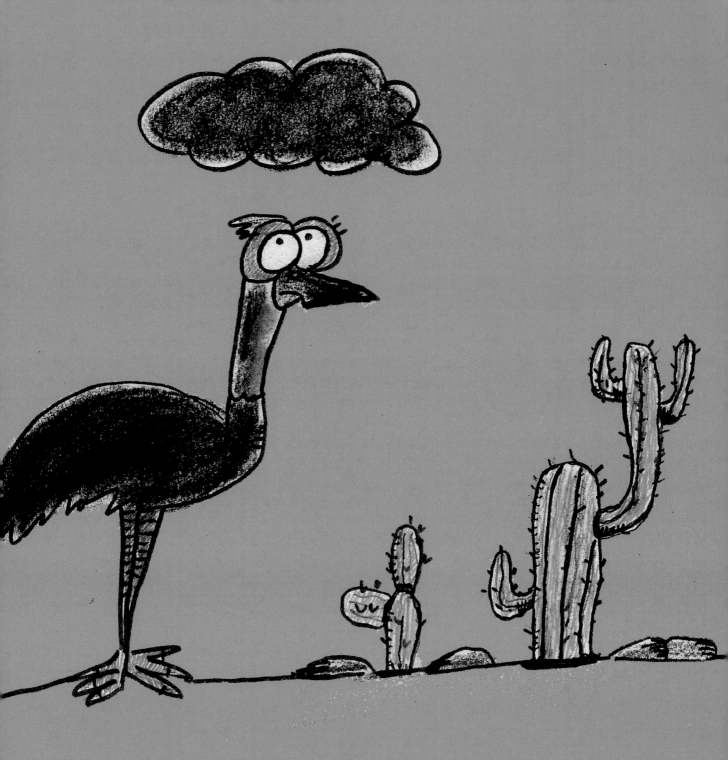

I felt really LONLEY. The dark cloud over my head doesn't *seem* to go away.

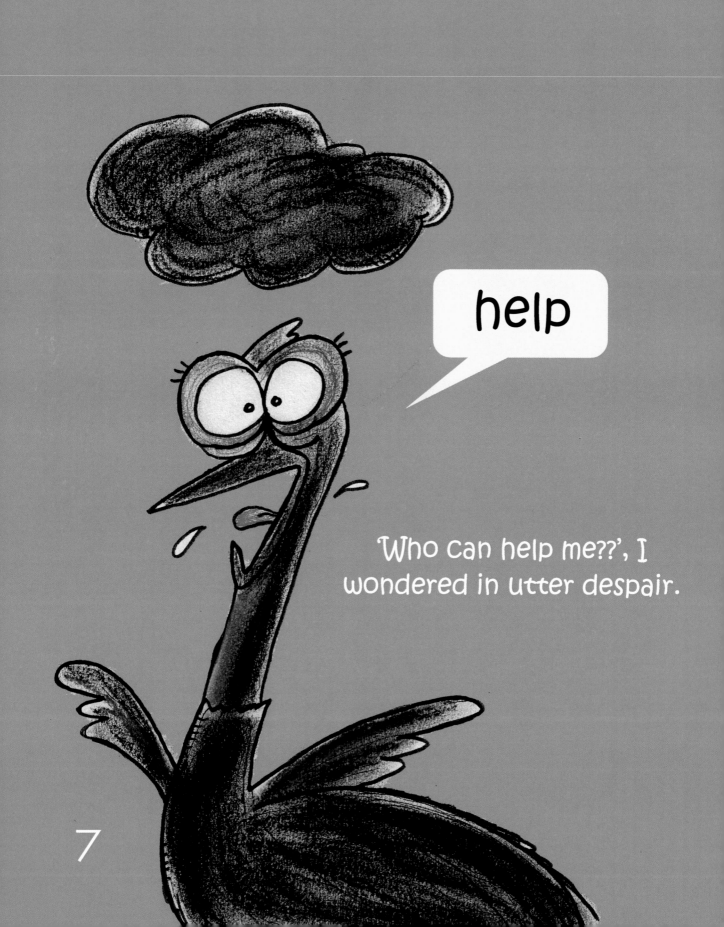

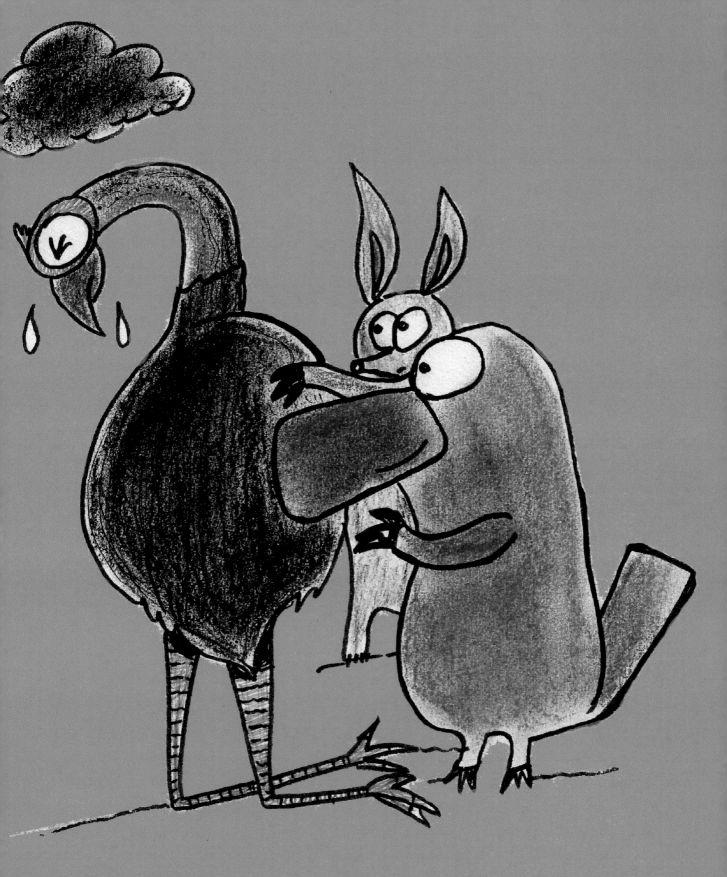

I felt a tap on my bum. It was my best mates
Isina the bilby and Plato the platypus.

I pulled my head out from under the pillow.

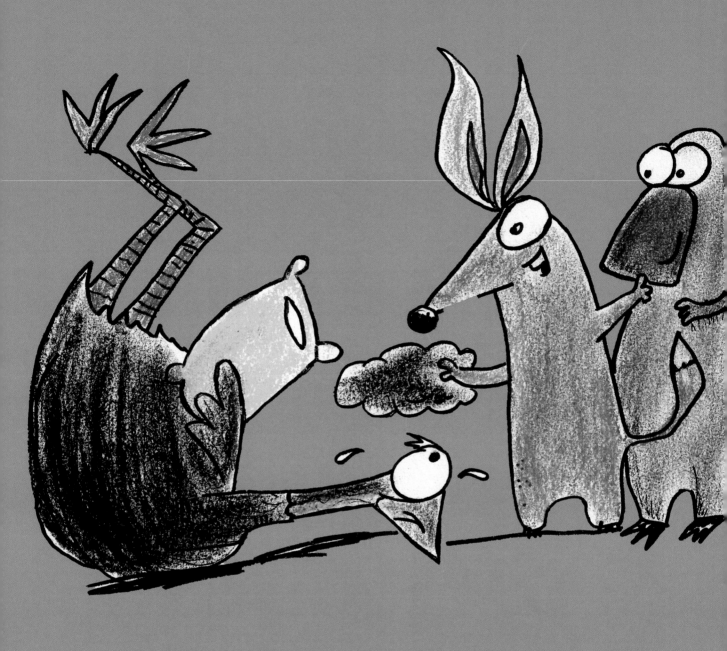

We were all trying to talk to you. But you seemed to be too carried away by your sadness, with your head buried under the pillow', said Isina.

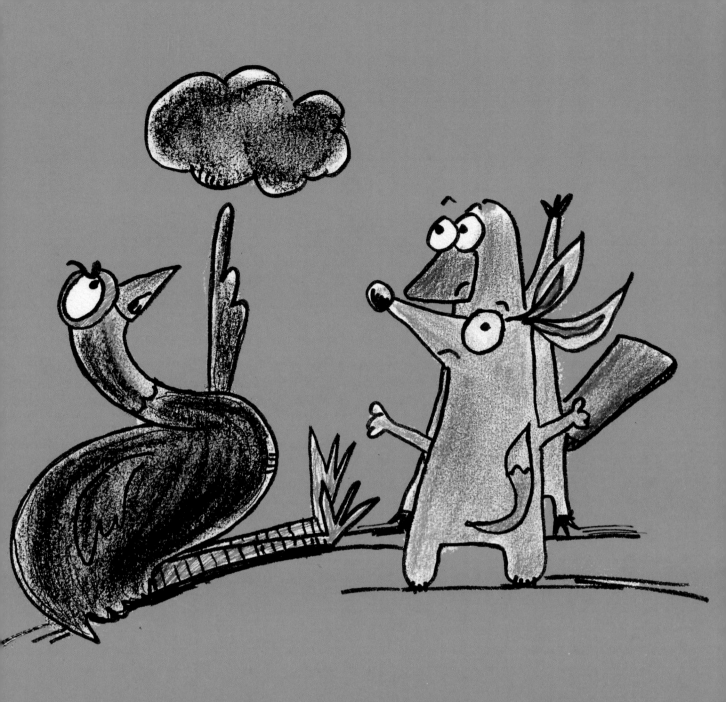

'I was so sad with this dark cloud over my head. I wish it went away', replied Georgina.

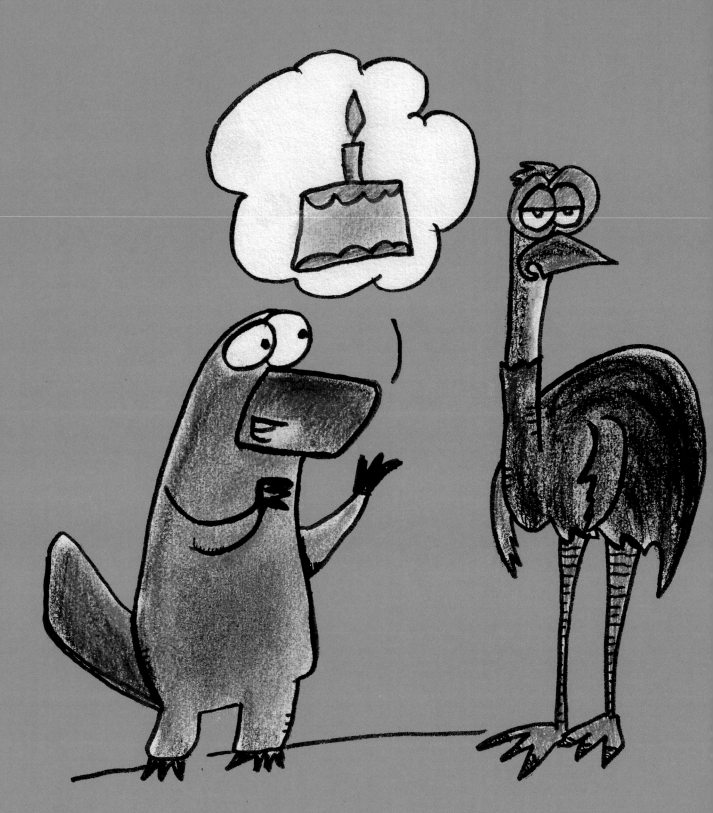

'We didn't see you for footy. We didn't see you for Jayena's birthday party either!

We were worried what was happening to you', asked Plato concerned.

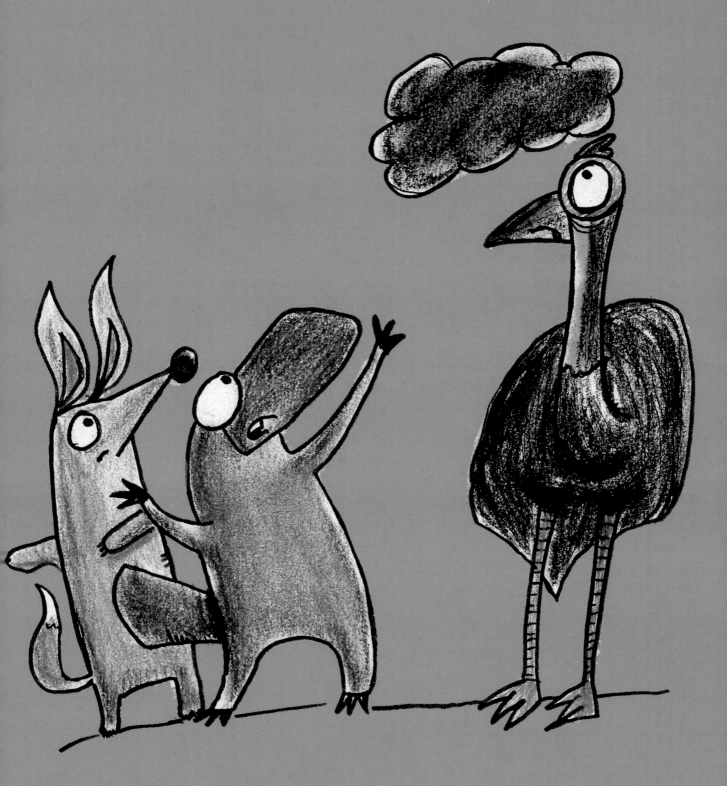

'By the way how did you get this dark cloud over your head', asked Plato curiously.

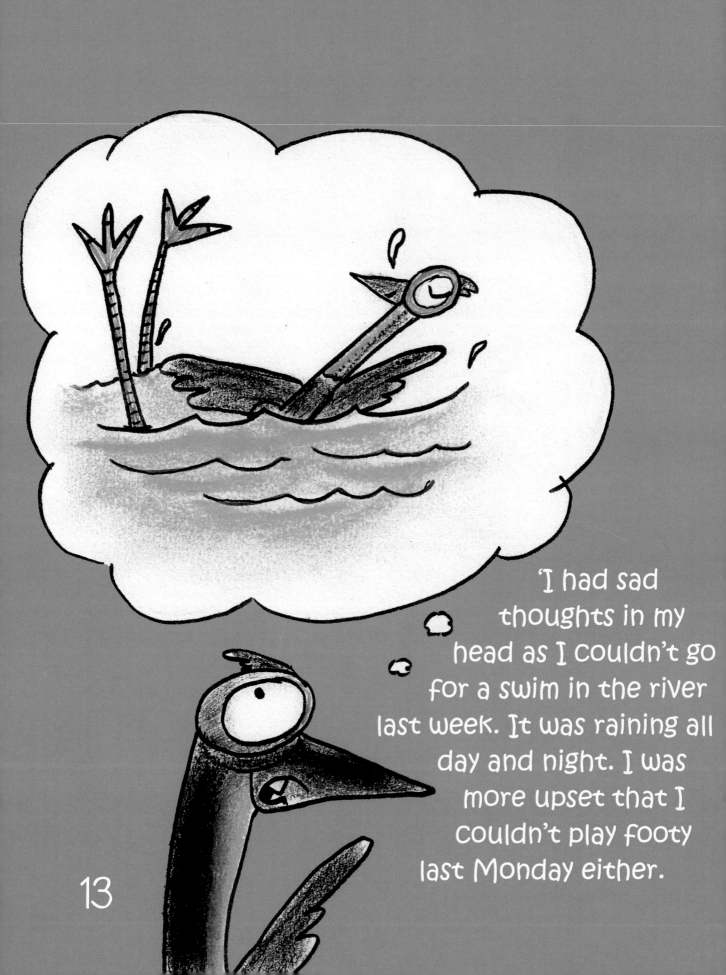

'I had sad thoughts in my head as I couldn't go for a swim in the river last week. It was raining all day and night. I was more upset that I couldn't play footy last Monday either.

13

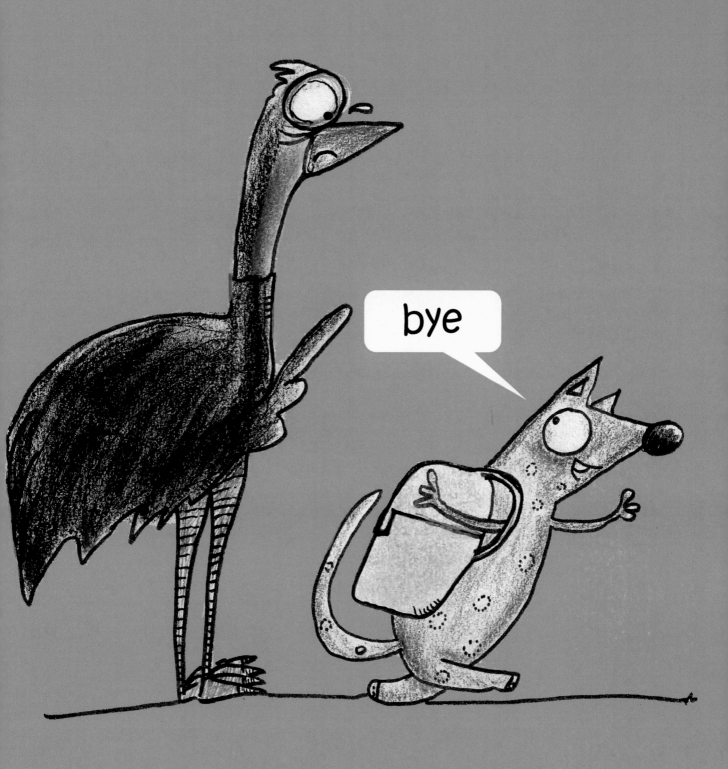

I felt totally miserable that our best friend Tisy, the quoll left for another school last week.

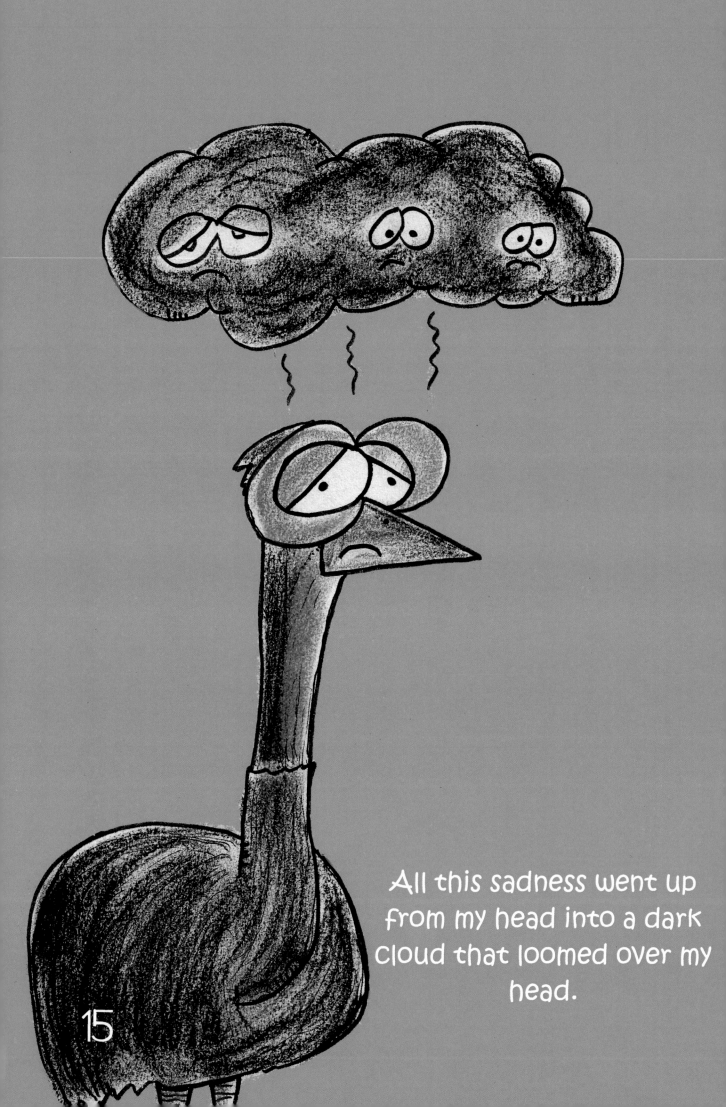

All this sadness went up from my head into a dark cloud that loomed over my head.

15

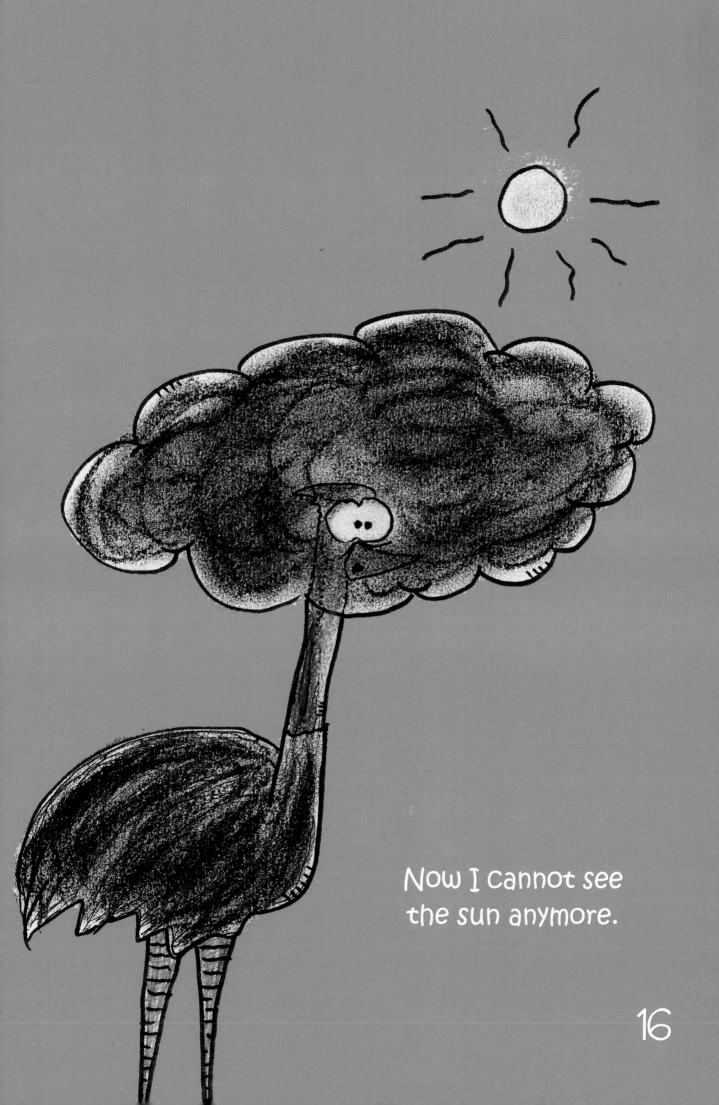

Now I cannot see
the sun anymore.

16

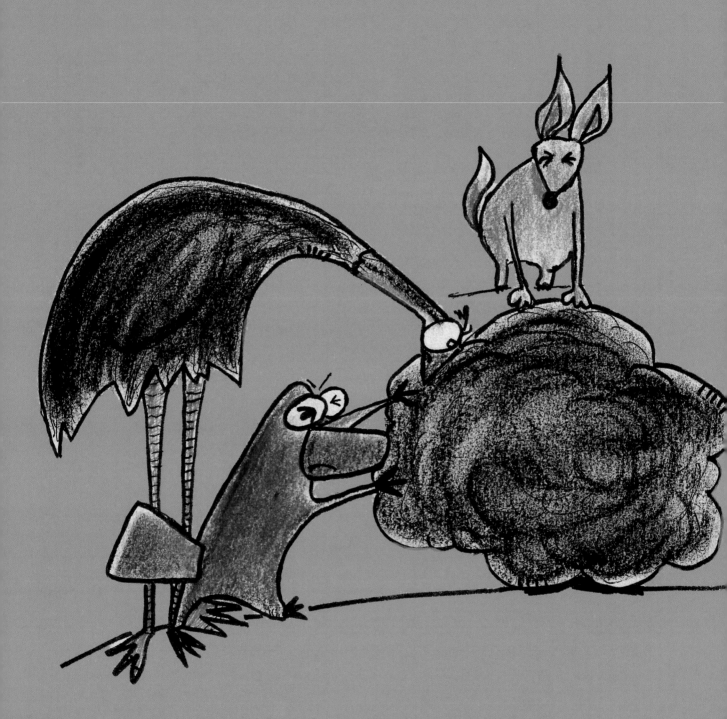

'So let us help you clear this DARK CLOUD over your head Georgina. How about we all go for a swim in the river together right now?

17

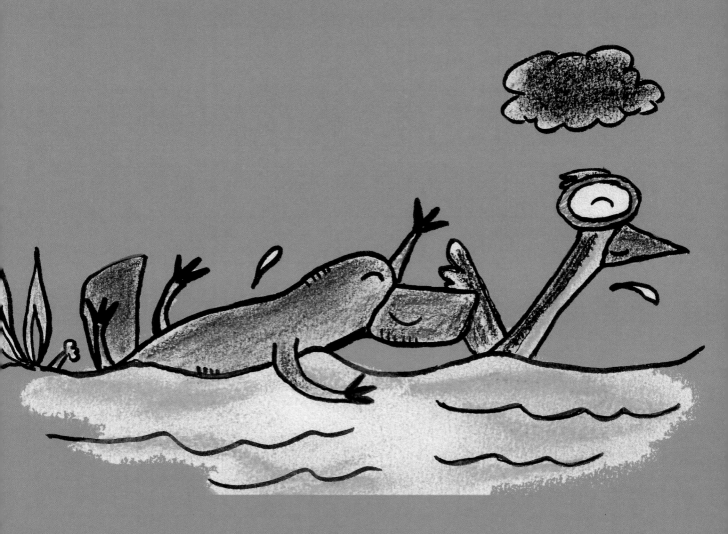

As they were swimming together, the dark cloud over Georgina's head seemed to shrink.

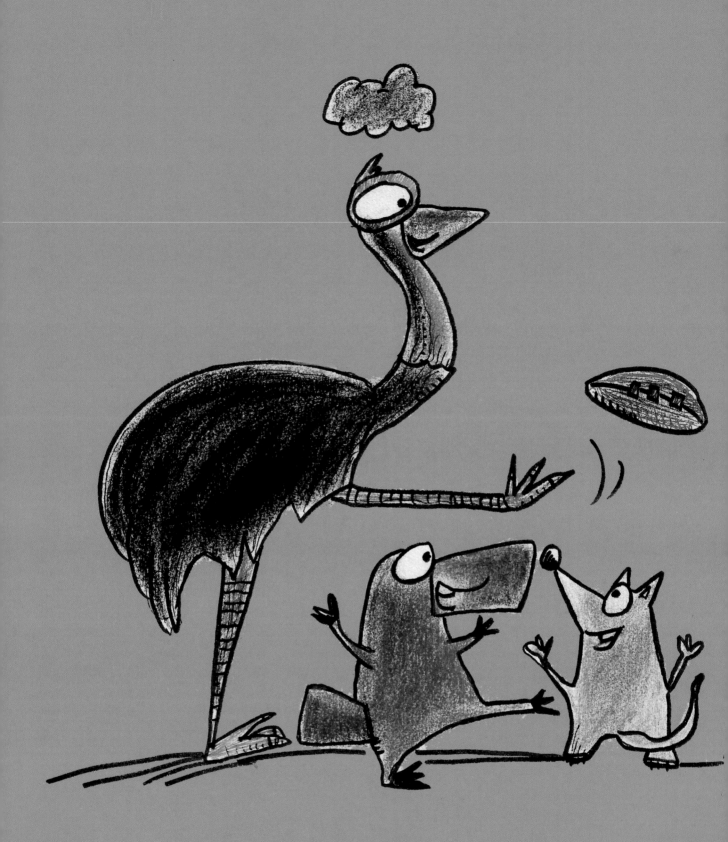

'It has stopped raining today, let us go out for a game of footy', said Isina. The dark cloud over Georgina's head got even smaller when the friends finished the footy game.

19

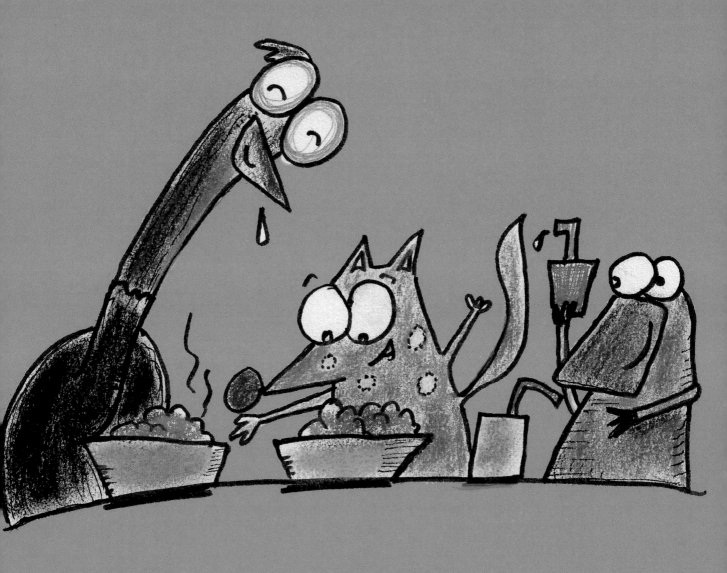

'Let us give a good farewell party to Tisy, who is leaving our school to have a greater opportunity at the new school', said Plato.

20

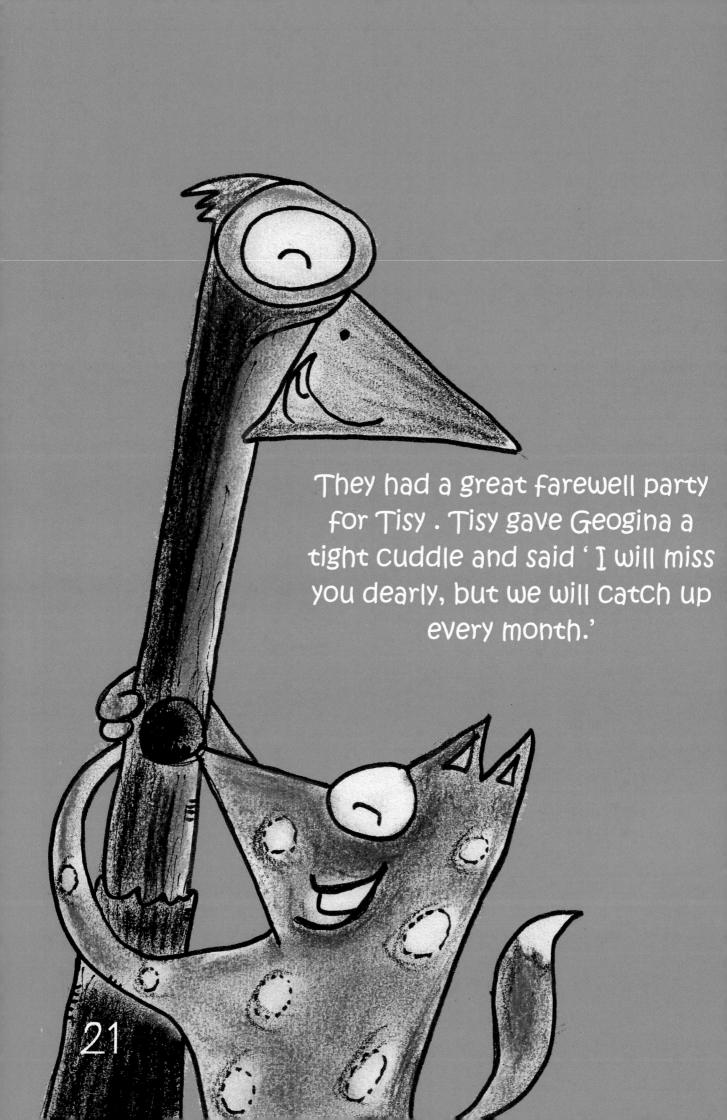

They had a great farewell party for Tisy . Tisy gave Geogina a tight cuddle and said ' I will miss you dearly, but we will catch up every month.'

21

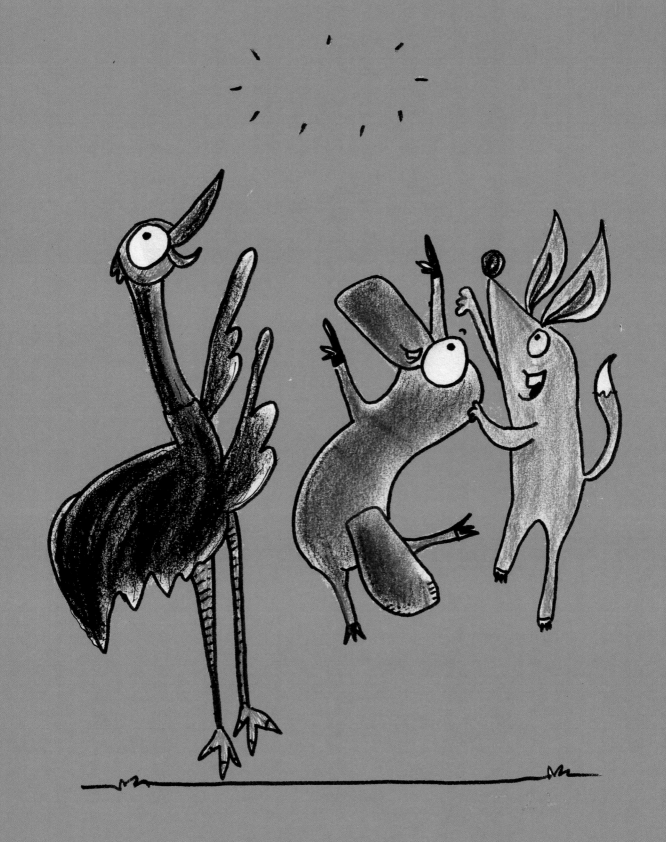

At the end of the party Georgina looked up and screamed in delight.' Hurray!!! The dark cloud over my head has disappeared!'

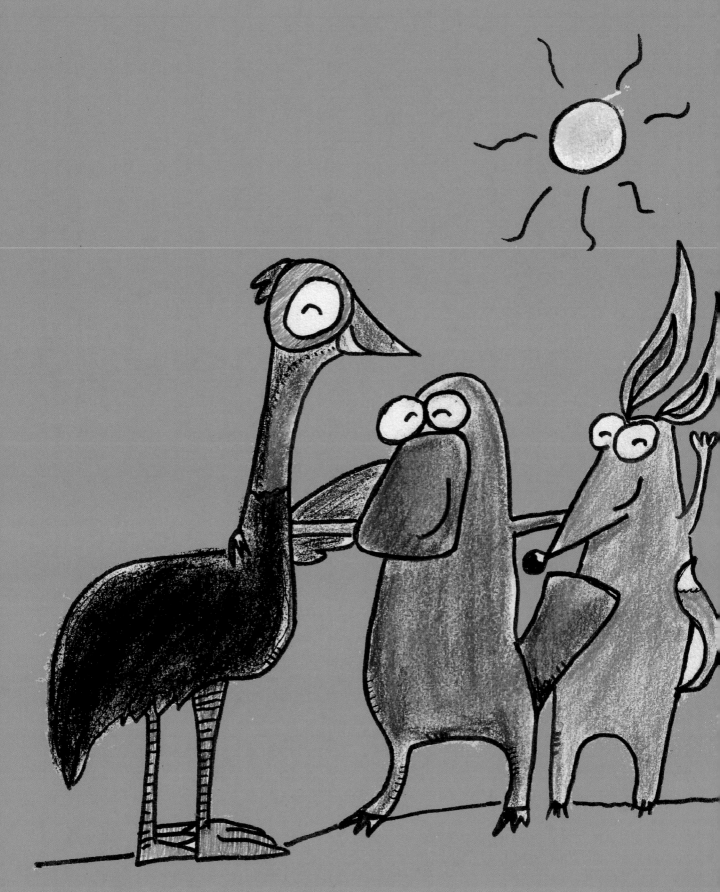

I can see sun now and I feel HAPPY
again. Thankyou all!

23

'It is ok to have dark thoughts on and off Georgina, but we will all help each other to get rid of it. Please don't stick your head under the pillow and cry when you have friends around you who can make you feel better dear . We are all here to help.' Plato smiled and said.

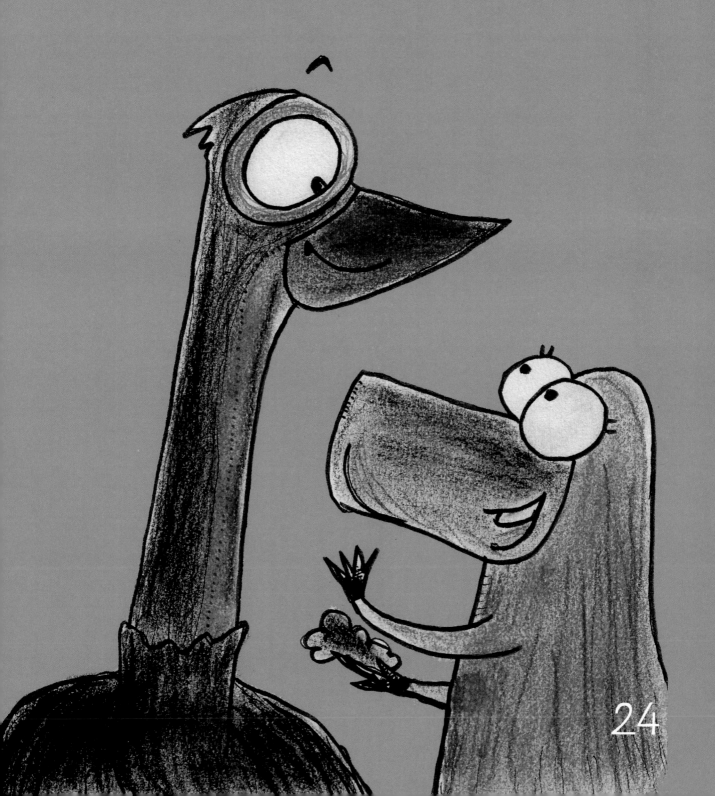

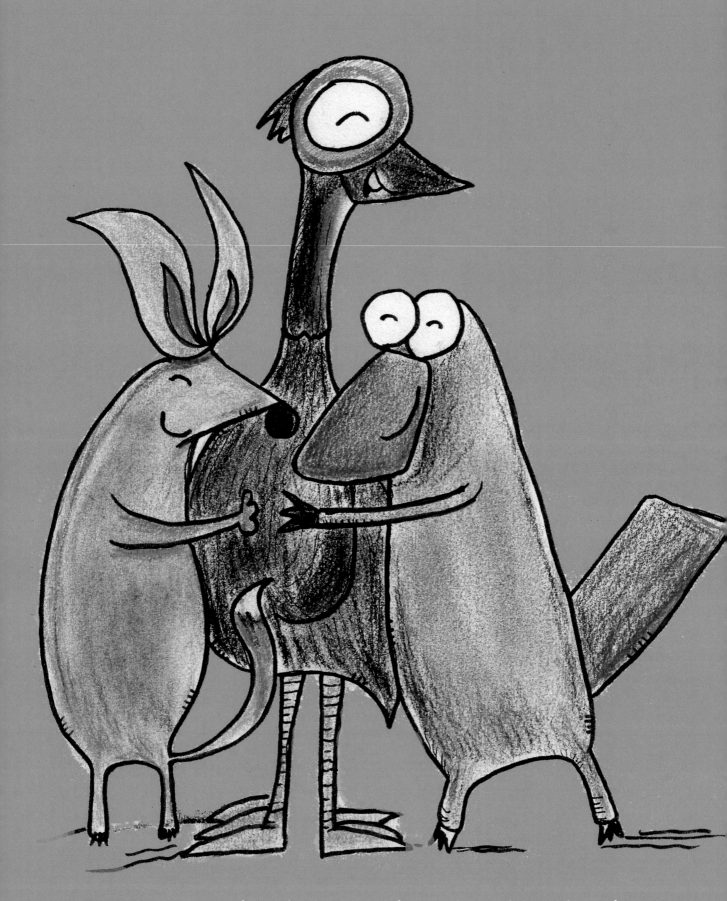

The friends hugged each other, held
each other's hands and walked down
the path together.

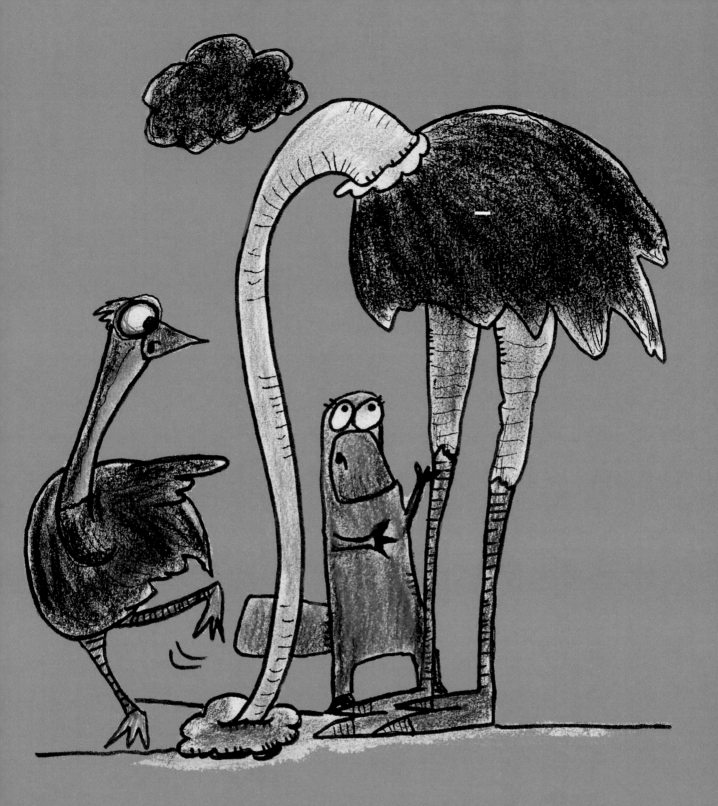

Soon they came across Zon, the ostrich with a dark cloud over her head. She had her head buried under the ground and was sobbing.

"Oops, looks like she needs help too'. Saying this they all ran up to Zon to help her out.

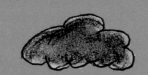

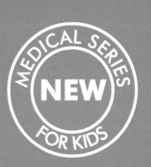

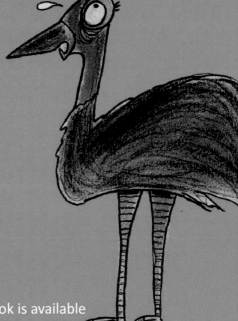

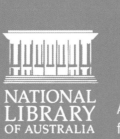

Made in the USA
Las Vegas, NV
15 September 2021